Migraine Relief Kitchen: Delicious Recipes for Migraine Management

by

Nancy M. Smith

Table of Contents

Introduction: Migraine Relief Through Diet

Migraines, those crippling and often terrible headaches, can sometimes be traced back to what we consume. Certain meals and dietary cues have been demonstrated in studies to provoke migraine attacks. These triggers may differ from person to person, making it critical for migraine patients to identify their dietary culprits.

Foods like aged cheeses, processed meats, chocolate, and alcohol are all major migraine triggers. Additionally, chemicals such as monosodium glutamate (MSG) and the artificial sweetener aspartame have been linked to migraine attacks in sensitive individuals.

Individuals can greatly lessen the frequency and severity of their migraines by understanding these dietary linkages and implementing a migraine-friendly diet. This book will walk you through the process, giving you tasty recipes and helpful tips on how to turn your kitchen into a migraine-relief sanctuary.

The major purpose of this cookbook is to provide you with a treasure trove of tasty dishes customized exclusively to help you manage and prevent migraines. We recognize the difficulties that migraine sufferers endure, and one key component of this difficulty is making the appropriate food choices.

The recipes in this book have been thoughtfully created with your health in mind. They lessen the chance of migraine attacks because they are free of known migraine triggers and are made to be easy on your system. Our mission is to provide you with a pleasurable and healthy eating experience so you can enjoy your food without having to worry about always getting a migraine.

Whether you're looking for a nutritious breakfast, a filling lunch, a tasty supper, or even snacks and sweet treats, we've got you covered. We're here to prove that a migraine-friendly diet doesn't have to be devoid of flavor or variety. By the end of this book, we hope you'll have a collection of recipes that not only satisfy your taste buds but also help you on your way to a migraine-free life.

1. **Blueberry Bliss Smoothie**: Start your day with this delicious and migraine-safe smoothie packed with antioxidants and natural sweetness.
2. **Quinoa Salad with Lemon Herb Dressing**: A delicious, easy-to-make salad that mixes quinoa, fresh vegetables, and a zesty dressing to satisfy your lunch needs.
3. **Herb-Roasted Fish**: A wonderful dinner choice containing luscious fish coupled with a blend of aromatic herbs, delivering a savory, migraine-friendly meal.
4. **Mango Tango Sorbet**: For a delicious treat, try this dairy-free sorbet brimming with the tropical taste of ripe mangoes.
5. **Crispy Baked Chickpeas**: A tasty and crispy snack to keep your energy levels up without jeopardizing your migraine-safe diet.

These are only a few of the delectable recipes you may find in this guidebook. To make sure you enjoy your meals while efficiently treating your migraines, we've carefully selected a selection of recipes. Prepare to enjoy these recipes without having to worry about bringing on a migraine, and learn how having a migraine-friendly kitchen may make your life easier.

Chapter 1: The Crucial Migraine Diet

Principles of a Migraine-Friendly Diet

Following some fundamental guidelines intended to reduce migraine triggers and enhance general well-being is part of developing a diet that is gentle on your brain and heart. The following guidelines form the foundation of your migraine relief kitchen:

1. **Fresh and Whole Foods**: Whenever possible, choose foods that are fresh and unprocessed. Your meals should be centered around whole grains, lean proteins, and an abundance of fruits and vegetables.

2. **Low Tyramine**: Some people experience migraines when they consume tyramine, which is present in some foods, including aged cheeses and cured meats. Eat fewer or none of these foods high in tyramine.

3. **Hydration**: Headaches may result from dehydration. Make sure you drink lots of water to stay well-hydrated throughout the day.

4. **Moderate Caffeine**: Caffeine withdrawal can cause migraines, but excessive caffeine ingestion can also cause migraines. Determine the right balance for you.

5. **Balanced Meals**: Aim for meals that are well-balanced in terms of protein, complex carbs, and healthy fats. This balance helps to normalize blood sugar levels, lowering the likelihood of headaches.

6. **Mindful Eating**: Eat your meals deliberately, paying attention to the flavors, textures, and emotions elicited by the food. This exercise can assist you in identifying and dealing with potential triggers.

7. **Eating Regularly**: Skipping meals can result in low blood sugar, which is a known migraine cause. Maintain

consistent meal times and, if necessary, include nutritious snacks.

8. **Limit Food Additives**: Certain food additives, such as monosodium glutamate (MSG), can cause migraines. Read food labels carefully and choose additive-free options.

9. **Personalize Your Diet**: Keep in mind that migraine triggers differ from person to person. Pay heed to your body's cues and adjust your diet accordingly.

Typical Migraine Triggers to Prevent

Migraines can be brought on by several factors, including eating habits. To reduce your risk of migraine attacks, it's critical to be aware of and avoid the following common migraine triggers:

- **Aged Cheeses**: Certain cheeses, such as blue cheese, cheddar, and Parmesan, contain tyramine, which is known to aggravate migraines. Choose fresh cheeses such as mozzarella or cottage cheese.

- **Processed Meats**: Nitrites and nitrates, which can cause migraines in certain people, are commonly found in cold cuts, bacon, and hot dogs. Choose unprocessed, fresh meats.
- **Caffeine**: While caffeine withdrawal can cause headaches, excessive caffeine use can also be harmful. Monitor your caffeine intake and avoid abrupt changes to your caffeine schedule.
- **Alcohol**: Red wine, beer, and specific spirits such as whiskey and champagne are major migraine triggers. If you prefer to consume alcohol, do so in moderation.
- **Artificial Sweeteners**: Aspartame and other artificial sweeteners have been connected to migraines in some people. Choose natural sweeteners like honey or stevia.
- **Salty Foods**: High-sodium foods can contribute to dehydration, which can be a

migraine trigger. Reduce your intake of salty snacks and processed foods.

- **Monosodium Glutamate (MSG)**: MSG, a flavor enhancer found in many manufactured and restaurant foods, has been associated with migraines. Read food labels and select MSG-free products.
- **Food Additives**: Certain food additives, such as sulfites and food colors, have been linked to migraines. Seek foods that are free of these substances.
- **Tyramine-Rich Foods**: Tyramine-rich foods such as pickles, sauerkraut, and soy sauce can be harmful for some people. Limit your intake of these foods.
- **Chocolate**: While it's a popular delicacy, chocolate includes both caffeine and tyramine, which can cause migraines. White chocolate or carob are good substitutes.
- **Nuts and Seeds**: Peanuts, cashews, and certain seeds, such as sunflower seeds, can be rich in tyramine. Choose low-tyramine

alternatives such as almonds or pumpkin seeds.

- **Citrus Fruits**: Oranges, lemons, and limes are acidic and might cause migraines in some people. Consider different fruits, such as apples and pears.

By being aware of these frequent migraine triggers and making wise dietary choices, you can lower the likelihood of migraine attacks and strive toward improved headache management.

Quick Start Guide for Your Migraine-Friendly Diet

It's not too hard to start eating in a way that will help with migraines. To assist you in beginning the process of controlling your migraines with a diet, consider the following brief advice:

- **Keep a Food Diary**: Before making any dietary adjustments, start by monitoring your meals and migraine episodes. This will aid you in identifying your triggers and tendencies.

- **Gradual Modifications**: Instead of changing your diet all at once, start with small modifications. In the long run, gradually substitute migraine-friendly diets for trigger foods.
- **Maintain Hydration**: Dehydration is a typical migraine trigger. To stay hydrated, drink plenty of water throughout the day.
- **Balance Your Meals**: Aim for balanced meals that include lean protein, complete grains, and plenty of fruits and vegetables. Balanced meals can help balance blood sugar levels and lessen migraine risk.
- **Restrict Processed Meals**: Processed meals frequently contain additives and preservatives that may contribute to migraines. When possible, select fresh, whole foods.
- **Read Labels**: Read food labels carefully to look for potential migraine triggers such as MSG, artificial sweeteners, and sulfites.

- **Moderate Caffeine**: If you are a regular caffeine user, avoid abrupt withdrawal, which can cause headaches. If necessary, gradually reduce caffeine consumption.
- **Cook at Home**: Preparing meals at home allows you to have more control over the ingredients and cooking procedures. It's an efficient method for avoiding migraine triggers.
- **Plan and Prep**: Plan your meals ahead of time and do some meal prep to ensure you have migraine-friendly options on hand.
- **Consult with a Dietitian**: If you require personalized guidance or are confused about your food choices, it is advisable to speak with a qualified dietitian who specializes in migraine treatment.

Recall that it could take some time before you make substantial dietary adjustments to reduce the frequency and intensity of your migraines. Try to recognize and stay away from your triggers, but be patient and persistent in your efforts.

Chapter 2: Easy Breakfast to Prepare

Delectable Breakfast Ideas That Are Migraine-Friendly

A healthy and migraine-friendly breakfast might help you have a migraine-free day. Here are a few simple breakfast recipes that are kind to your head:

Berry Blast Smoothie

Ingredients:

- 1 cup mixed berries (blueberries, strawberries, raspberries)
- 1 banana
- 1/2 cup plain Greek yogurt
- 1 tbsp. Honey (optional)
- 1/2 cup almond milk

Instructions:

- Wash the mixed berries (blueberries, strawberries, and raspberries).

- Peel and slice the banana.
- Measure out the plain Greek yogurt, honey (if using), and almond milk.
- Blend the mixed berries, sliced banana, plain Greek yogurt, honey (if using), and almond milk in a blender.
- Blend the ingredients on high until smooth and creamy. You can modify the thickness by adding more or less almond milk to your liking.
- Taste the smoothie and adjust the sweetness with more honey if necessary.
- Transfer the smoothie into a glass or a travel-friendly container.
- Serve your wonderful "Berry Blast Smoothie" immediately and enjoy!

Avocado Toast

Ingredients:

- 1 ripe avocado
- 2 slices whole-grain bread
- 1 small tomato, sliced
- Salt and pepper to taste

Instructions:

- Slice the mature avocado in half, extract the flesh from the pit, and transfer it to a bowl.
- Mash the avocado with a fork until it reaches the desired creaminess.
- Slice off the small tomato.
- Toast the two slices of whole-grain bread until crisp and brown.
- Take some toasted, whole-grain bread slices.
- Distribute the mashed avocado evenly on each slice.
- Arrange the tomato slices on top of the avocado spread.
- Season the tomato slices with a touch of salt and a splash of pepper.
- Your avocado toast is now ready to serve! Serve on a dish and enjoy the creamy avocado, juicy tomatoes, and crunch of whole-grain bread.

Overnight Oats

Ingredients:

- 1/2 cup oats, old-fashioned
- 1/2 cup of almond milk
- 1/2 cup diced fresh fruit (apple, pear, or berry)
- 1 tbsp. Honey (optional)

Instructions:

- Combine the old-fashioned oats and almond milk in a lidded container or jar. Mix them until well blended.
  Add the diced fresh fruit of your choosing. You can use apples, pears, berries, or any other fruit you like.
  If you like your oats sweeter, sprinkle one tablespoon of honey over the oats and fruit. This stage is optional and can be modified to suit your tastes.
  Stir together all of the ingredients in the container until fully combined.
  Refrigerate the container with a lid. Allow the mixture to set and chill overnight, or for at least 4-6 hours.

Remove the container from the refrigerator the next morning or whenever you're ready to eat.

- To ensure that everything is well incorporated, give the overnight oats a thorough toss.
- The overnight oats can be eaten straight out of the container or transferred to a bowl for serving.
- If desired, decorate with more fruit or nuts.
- It's time to enjoy your nourishing and tasty overnight oats. This is a fantastic choice for a nutritious and expedient breakfast that can be had at your convenience.

Scrambled Eggs with Spinach

Ingredients:

- 2 eggs
- 1 cup fresh spinach, chopped
- 1/4 cup diced bell peppers
- Salt and pepper to taste

Instructions:

- 2 eggs, cracked into a bowl, beaten with a fork or whisk until the yolks and whites are well mixed.
  Cut the fresh spinach and dice the bell peppers. You can use any hue of bell pepper you choose.
  Heat a nonstick skillet or frying pan over medium heat.
  Once the pan is hot, add the diced bell peppers. You can use a small quantity of cooking spray or a drop of oil if you want.
  Sauté the bell peppers for a few minutes, or until they soften and turn somewhat brown.
  Add the fresh spinach to the pan. Stir and cook for another 1-2 minutes, or until the spinach has wilted.
- To taste, add a pinch of salt and pepper to the vegetables. Note that eggs can also have a naturally salty taste, so watch the salt.

- Pour the whisked eggs onto the skillet of sautéed veggies.
- Mix the eggs with the sautéed vegetables after gently scrambling them with a spatula. The eggs should be thoroughly cooked but still soft and a little moist, so keep cooking and stirring.
- When the scrambled eggs are done to your satisfaction, move them to a platter.
  It's time to enjoy your scrambled eggs with spinach. Greens and protein abound in this satisfying and appetizing meal.

Greek Yogurt Parfait

Ingredients:

- 1 cup Greek yogurt
- 1/2 cup granola (look for options without added triggers)
- 1/2 cup mixed fresh fruit (e.g., bananas, strawberries)

Instructions:

- Make sure you have all of the following components ready: 1 cup Greek yogurt, 1/2 cup granola (select a variety without additional migraine triggers), and 1/2 cup mixed fresh fruit, such as bananas and strawberries.
- Begin by grabbing a glass or a dish. Spoon a layer of Greek yogurt into the bottom of the container.
- Top with granola. Choose a granola variation that doesn't contain any migraine-inducing elements based on your dietary choices.
- Place a layer of mixed fresh fruit on top of the granola. You can use sliced bananas, halved strawberries, or any other fruit you like.
- If you want a larger parfait or additional layers, repeat the process by adding another layer of Greek yogurt, granola, and fresh fruit.
- Finish your parfait with an extra layer of fresh fruit on top. It offers a lovely splash of color and taste.

- Your Greek yogurt parfait is ready to serve. It's a tasty and healthy snack or breakfast. The creamy Greek yogurt, crunchy granola, and sweet fresh fruit make for a wonderful and filling combo.

Recall that avoiding possible triggers such as processed meals and artificial additives is the key to a migraine-friendly breakfast. These recipes offer a healthy, well-balanced breakfast without compromising on taste. Take pleasure in your mornings without fear of inducing a migraine.

Chapter 3: Healthy Lunches

Mouthwatering Lunch Ideas to Prevent Migraine

Making healthful, migraine-friendly meals is crucial to maintaining a balanced diet and reducing headache triggers when attempting to manage migraines. Here, we've compiled a list of mouthwatering lunch ideas that will both quench your hunger and prevent migraines.

Grilled Chicken and Quinoa Salad

Ingredients:

- 2 boneless, skinless chicken breasts
- 1 cup quinoa
- 2 cups water
- 2 tablespoons olive oil
- 1 teaspoon paprika
- 1 teaspoon garlic powder
- Salt and black pepper to taste
- 6 cups mixed salad greens
- 1 cup cherry tomatoes, halved

- 1/2 cucumber, sliced
- 1/4 red onion, thinly sliced
- 1/4 cup balsamic vinaigrette dressing

Instructions:

- Preheat your grill to medium-high heat.
- Olive oil, paprika, garlic powder, salt, and black pepper should all be combined in a mixing bowl.
- Brush the chicken breasts with the olive oil and spice mixture.
- Grill the chicken for about 6-7 minutes per side, or until it's thoroughly done and has excellent grill marks. The chicken should be cooked through to 165°F (74°C). Remove the chicken from the grill and set it aside for a few minutes to rest. It should be cut into strips.
- While the chicken is roasting, rinse the quinoa with cold water. Place the quinoa in a pot with water. Bring to a boil, then reduce to a low heat, cover, and simmer for about 15 minutes, or until the quinoa is cooked and the water has been absorbed.

Take off from the heat source and let it cool.

- Mix the cooked quinoa, mixed salad greens, cherry tomatoes, cucumber, and red onion in a large mixing bowl.
- Drizzle the dressing over the salad.
- On top, arrange the grilled and sliced chicken.
- Toss everything carefully to combine.
- Your Grilled Chicken and Quinoa Salad is now ready to serve as a nutritional and migraine-friendly lunch choice. Enjoy!

Vegetable Stir-Fry with Brown Rice

Ingredients:

- 2 cups cooked brown rice
- 2 tablespoons vegetable oil
- 1 small onion, thinly sliced
- 2 cloves garlic, minced
- 1 red bell pepper, sliced
- 1 yellow bell pepper, sliced
- 1 cup broccoli florets
- 1 cup snap peas

- 1 carrot, julienned
- 1/4 cup low-sodium soy sauce
- 2 tablespoons rice vinegar
- 1 tablespoon honey (optional)
- 1 teaspoon fresh ginger, grated
- 1/2 teaspoon red pepper flakes (modify according to taste)
- Salt and black pepper to taste
- Chopped green onions for garnish

Instructions:

- The vegetable oil should be heated over medium-high heat in a large skillet or wok.
- Simmer the onions for 2 to 3 minutes, or until they start to get tender.
- Cook for 30 seconds more, or until the minced garlic is aromatic.
- Stir in the red and yellow bell peppers, broccoli florets, snap peas, and julienned carrots. The vegetables should be stir-fried for 5 to 7 minutes, or until they are crisp-tender.

- In a small bowl, combine the soy sauce, rice vinegar, honey (if using), grated ginger, and red pepper flakes. Pour this sauce over the vegetables.
- Stir carefully to evenly coat the vegetables with the sauce. Cook for an additional 2-3 minutes, or until everything is well cooked.
- Add salt and pepper to taste. To suit your tastes, add or subtract seasoning.
- Arrange the cooked brown rice on a serving platter, then spoon the stir-fried vegetables over it.
- Chopped green onions are a nice garnish.
- You can now enjoy a tasty and migraine-friendly meal of your vegetable stir-fry with brown rice.

Spinach and Feta Stuffed Chicken Breast:

Ingredients:

- 2 boneless, skinless chicken breasts
- 2 cups fresh spinach leaves
- 1/2 cup crumbled feta cheese

- 1/4 cup sun-dried tomatoes, chopped
- 2 cloves garlic, minced
- 1 tablespoon olive oil
- 1/2 teaspoon dried oregano
- 1/2 teaspoon dried basil
- Salt and black pepper to taste
- Toothpicks or kitchen twine for securing

Instructions:

- Preheat your oven to 375°F (190°C). Warm the olive oil in a pan over medium heat. Cook for 30 seconds, or until the garlic is spicy.
- In the skillet, add the fresh spinach leaves. Sauté for 2-3 minutes, or until wilted and reduced in volume. Season with salt and pepper to taste.
- Turn off the heat and set the skillet aside to cool for a few minutes.
- While the spinach is cooling, butterfly each chicken breast. This means you'll cut each breast almost all the way through, so you can open it like a book.

- Half the sautéed spinach should be placed on one side of each butterflied chicken breast. Garnish the spinach with crumbled feta cheese and sliced sun-dried tomatoes.
- Sprinkle dry oregano and basil over the fillings.
- Close the chicken breasts over the fillings, fastening them with toothpicks or kitchen twine to keep the fillings in place.
- Season the outside of each packed chicken breast with oregano, basil, salt, and black pepper.
- Place the packed chicken breasts on a baking sheet and bake for 25-30 minutes, or until the chicken is cooked through and no longer pink in the center. The cooking time will vary based on the thickness of your chicken breasts.
- Remove the toothpicks or string from the chicken once it has finished cooking.
- Serve your Spinach and Feta Stuffed Chicken Breast with your choice of side dishes or a light salad.

- Enjoy your wonderful and migraine-friendly meal!

Salmon Avocado Wrap

Ingredients:

- 2 whole-wheat tortillas or wraps
- 2 salmon fillets, grilled and flaked
- 1 ripe avocado, sliced
- 1/2 cup cherry tomatoes, halved
- 1/4 cup red onion, thinly sliced
- 2 cups fresh spinach leaves
- 2 tablespoons Greek yogurt (or a migraine-friendly dressing of your choice)
- Salt and black pepper to taste

Instructions:

- Begin by grilling the salmon fillets until they are fully done. This normally takes about 4-5 minutes per side, although cooking time will vary depending on the thickness of the fillets. Season the salmon with salt and black pepper while grilling.

- Once the salmon is cooked, flake it into smaller pieces.
- Place the whole-wheat tortillas or wraps on a sanitized surface.
- Spread a dollop of Greek yogurt or your chosen migraine-friendly dressing on each tortilla.
- Place a cup of fresh spinach leaves on top of each tortilla's dressing.
- Arrange the grilled and flaked fish on the spinach leaves.
- Arrange the sliced avocado, cherry tomatoes, and red onion evenly on top of the salmon.
- For more taste, season with a small teaspoon of salt and a little black pepper.
- Gently coil the tortillas, ensuring the edges are tucked in, to create a wrap.
- The wraps are now prepared for consumption; just cut them in half if preferred.
- A tasty and migraine-friendly lunch option is these salmon avocado wraps. Take pleasure in it!

Mediterranean Quinoa Bowl

Ingredients:

- 1 cup quinoa
- 2 cups water
- 1 can (15 ounces) washed and drained chickpeas
- 1 cup cherry tomatoes, halved
- 1 cucumber, diced
- 1/2 red onion, finely chopped
- 1/2 cup Kalamata olives, pitted and sliced
- 1/4 cup fresh parsley, chopped
- 1/4 cup fresh mint leaves, chopped
- 3 tablespoons extra-virgin olive oil
- 2 tablespoons lemon juice
- 1 teaspoon ground cumin
- Salt and black pepper to taste

Instructions:

- To begin, carefully rinse the quinoa in cool water.
- Place the washed quinoa and water in a medium saucepan. Bring it to a boil, then

reduce the heat, cover, and leave it to simmer for about 15 minutes, or until the quinoa has absorbed the water and is soft. Allow to cool after removing from the heat.

- In a large mixing bowl, add the cooked and cooled quinoa, chickpeas, cherry tomatoes, cucumber, red onion, Kalamata olives, fresh parsley, and mint leaves.
- In a separate small bowl, whisk together the extra-virgin olive oil, lemon juice, ground cumin, salt, and black pepper to make a dressing.
- Drizzle the dressing over the quinoa mixture and toss until fully incorporated.
- Serve the Mediterranean Quinoa Bowl in individual bowls or on a plate.
- This Mediterranean-inspired quinoa bowl is a tasty and nutritious lunch alternative that is good for migraine prevention. Enjoy!

Black Bean and Sweet Potato Chili

Ingredients:

- 1 tablespoon olive oil
- 1 onion, chopped
- 2 cloves garlic, minced
- 1 red bell pepper, chopped
- 1 sweet potato, peeled and diced
- 2 teaspoons chili powder
- 1 teaspoon ground cumin
- 1/2 teaspoon paprika
- 1/2 teaspoon dried oregano
- 1 can (15 oz.) washed and drained black beans
- 1 can (14 ounces) diced tomatoes
- 2 cups vegetable broth
- Salt and black pepper to taste
- Fresh cilantro, chopped (for garnish)
- Avocado slices (for garnish)
- Lime wedges (for garnish)

Instructions:

- In a big pot, preheat the olive oil over medium heat.
- Add the chopped onion and simmer until transparent, about 5 minutes.

- Once fragrant, simmer for an additional minute after adding the minced garlic.
- Add the diced sweet potato and chopped red bell pepper to the saucepan. Cook until the sweet potato starts to soften, stirring periodically, for about 5 minutes.
- Add the dried oregano, paprika, chili powder, and ground cumin. Toss the veggies in the spices, coating them well.
- Add the vegetable broth, diced tomatoes (including juice), and drained black beans. Toss to blend.
- Add salt and black pepper to taste when preparing the chili. If you'd like, you can add more chili powder to change the degree of spice.
- Bring the mixture to a boil, then reduce the heat, cover, and leave to simmer for 20–25 minutes, or until the sweet potato is cooked.
- Serve the black bean and sweet potato chili in individual bowls, topped with chopped fresh cilantro, avocado slices, and lime wedges.

- This hearty and tasty chili is ideal for a migraine-friendly lunch. Enjoy!

Rice Noodle Salad with Shrimp:

Ingredients:

- 8 oz rice noodles
- 1 lb large shrimp, peeled and deveined
- 1 red bell pepper, thinly sliced
- 1 cucumber, julienned
- 2 carrots, julienned
- 3 green onions, chopped
- 1/4 cup fresh cilantro, chopped
- 1/4 cup fresh mint leaves, chopped
- 1/4 cup unsalted peanuts, chopped

For the Dressing:

- 3 tablespoons lime juice
- 2 tablespoons fish sauce
- 1 tablespoon brown sugar (adjust to taste)
- 1 clove garlic, minced
- 1/2 red chili, minced (adjust to taste)

Instructions:

- As directed on the package, prepare the rice noodles. To halt the cooking process, drain and rinse with cold water. Put away.

- Heat some oil in a big skillet over medium-high heat. Once the shrimp are added, fry them for two to three minutes on each side, or until they become opaque and pink. Take off the heat source and place it aside.

- The cooked rice noodles, cooked shrimp, sliced red bell pepper, julienned cucumber, carrots, chopped green onions, cilantro, and mint leaves should all be combined in a big bowl.

- To create the dressing, combine the lime juice, brown sugar, fish sauce, minced garlic, and minced red chile in a small bowl. To suit your tastes, adjust the amount of sweetness and spiciness.

- Make sure everything is thoroughly coated with the dressing by pouring the dressing over the salad components and tossing to mix.

- Present the rice noodle salad with shrimp in separate dishes, topped with chopped unsalted peanuts for crunch.
- This salad is a great option for a migraine-friendly lunch because it is delicious and refreshing. Pleasure yourself!

Chapter 4: Delicious Dinners

Making healthy, migraine-friendly dinners is crucial to keeping a balanced diet and reducing headache triggers when attempting to manage migraines. Here is a collection of mouthwatering dinner recipes that will tantalize your taste buds and avoid migraines.

Baked Salmon with Lemon-Dill Sauce:

Ingredients:

- 4 salmon fillets
- 2 tablespoons olive oil
- 2 tablespoons fresh dill, chopped
- Zest and juice of 1 lemon
- Salt and pepper to taste

Instructions:

- Set the oven temperature to 375°F, or 190°C.
- Arrange the salmon fillets on a sheet of parchment paper-lined baking pan.

- Combine the lemon zest, lemon juice, olive oil, fresh dill, salt, and pepper in a small bowl.
- Pour the mixture over the fillets of salmon.
- The salmon should flake easily with a fork after baking it in the preheated oven for 15 to 20 minutes.

Quinoa and Vegetable Stir-Fry

Ingredients:

- 1 cup quinoa
- 2 cups water or vegetable broth
- 2 tablespoons olive oil
- 1 red bell pepper, thinly sliced
- 1 zucchini, sliced
- 1 cup broccoli florets
- 1 cup snap peas
- 2 cloves garlic, minced
- 1/4 cup low-sodium soy sauce or tamari
- 2 tablespoons honey (adjust to taste)

Instructions:

- Rinse the quinoa thoroughly, then blend it with water or vegetable broth in a saucepan. Bring to a boil, then reduce to a low heat, cover, and cook for 15-20 minutes, or until the quinoa is fluffy and the liquid has been absorbed.
- Warm the olive oil in a large skillet or wok over medium-high heat.
- In the skillet, combine the red bell pepper, zucchini, broccoli, snap peas, and minced garlic. Stir-fry for 5-7 minutes, or until the vegetables are soft but still crunchy.
- To make the sauce, whisk together the soy sauce and honey in a small mixing dish.
- Pour the sauce over the stir-fried vegetables and simmer for a few minutes more.
- Serve the vegetable stir-fry over cooked quinoa.

Grilled Turkey with Mashed Sweet Potatoes

Ingredients:

- 4 turkey cutlets

- 2 tablespoons olive oil
- 1 teaspoon dried thyme
- 1/2 teaspoon garlic powder
- Salt and pepper to taste

For the Mashed Sweet Potatoes:

- 2 large sweet potatoes, peeled and diced
- 2 tablespoons butter (or dairy-free alternative)
- 1/4 cup milk (or dairy-free alternative)
- Salt and pepper to taste

Instructions:

- Turn the heat up to medium-high on your grill.
- Combine the olive oil, salt, pepper, garlic powder, and dried thyme in a small bowl.
- Apply this blend to the turkey cutlets.
- Cook on the grill for 4–5 minutes on each side, or until the turkey is thoroughly cooked.
- Sweet potatoes should be boiled until tender while the turkey is cooking. Shake

well, then mash in butter, milk, pepper, and salt.

- Present the grilled turkey with sweet potato mash on the side.

Lemon Herb Grilled Chicken

Ingredients:

- 4 boneless, skinless chicken breasts
- 2 tablespoons olive oil
- 2 cloves garlic, minced
- Zest and juice of 1 lemon
- 1 teaspoon dried thyme
- Salt and pepper to taste

Instructions:

- Set your grill's temperature to medium-high.
- Olive oil, garlic, lemon zest, lemon juice, dried thyme, salt, and pepper should all be combined in a bowl.
- Apply the mixture to the chicken breasts.

- Grill the chicken for 6 to 8 minutes on each side, or until it reaches 165°F (74°C) inside.

Vegetable and Lentil Curry

Ingredients:

- 1 cup red lentils
- 3 cups vegetable broth
- 2 tablespoons olive oil
- 1 onion, chopped
- 2 cloves garlic, minced
- 2 teaspoons curry powder
- 1 teaspoon ground cumin
- 1 teaspoon ground coriander
- 1 teaspoon turmeric
- 1 can (14 oz) diced tomatoes
- 2 cups mixed vegetables (e.g., carrots, bell peppers, green beans)

Instructions:

- Rinse the red lentils and mix them with the vegetable broth in a big pot. Bring to a boil, then reduce to a low heat and continue to cook for about 20 minutes, or until the lentils are mushy and the liquid has been absorbed.

- In a separate pan, heat the olive oil. Saute the onion and garlic until transparent.
- Mix in the curry powder, cumin, coriander, and turmeric.
- Cook until the vegetables are soft, then add the diced tomatoes and mixed vegetables.
- Stir in the cooked lentils and the veggie combination.
- Serve the vegetable and lentil curry as a filling meal.

Vegan Chickpea and Vegetable Stir-Fry

Ingredients:

- 1 can (15 oz) washed and drained chickpeas
- 2 cups mixed vegetables (e.g., bell peppers, broccoli, snap peas)
- 1/4 cup low-sodium soy sauce (gluten-free version: tamari)

- 2 tablespoons sesame oil
- 2 cloves garlic, minced
- 1 tablespoon fresh ginger, minced
- 2 cups cooked brown rice or quinoa

Instructions:

- Heat the sesame oil in a big pan over medium-high heat.
- After adding the garlic and ginger, simmer for one minute.
- Add the chickpeas and mixed veggies, and sauté for 5 to 7 minutes, or until the vegetables are soft.
- Add the tamari or low-sodium soy sauce and simmer for another two to three minutes.
- Serve with cooked quinoa or brown rice.

Grilled Salmon with Dill Sauce

- **For Pescatarian or Seafood Lovers**
- **Ingredients**:
- 4 salmon fillets
- 1 tablespoon olive oil

- Salt and pepper to taste
- Fresh dill for garnish
- **Dill Sauce**:
- 1/2 cup plain Greek yogurt
- 1 tablespoon fresh dill, chopped
- 1 tablespoon lemon juice
- 1 clove garlic, minced

Instructions:

- Set your grill's temperature to medium-high.
- Add salt and pepper to the salmon fillets after brushing them with olive oil.
- The salmon should flake easily with a fork after grilling it for about 4–5 minutes on each side.
- In a small bowl, combine the ingredients for the dill sauce while the salmon is grilling.
- Garnish the grilled salmon with fresh dill and serve it with a dab of dill sauce.

Chapter 5: Snacks & Sweet Bites

Healthy Migraine-Friendly Snack Ideas

Making healthy, migraine-friendly snacks is crucial to keeping a balanced diet and reducing headache triggers when attempting to manage migraines. Here is a collection of mouthwatering snack recipes that will tantalize your taste buds and avoid migraines.

Greek Yogurt with Honey and Berries:

Ingredients:

- 1 cup Greek yogurt
- 1 tbsp honey
- Fresh berries (strawberries, blueberries, raspberries) - Add a handful of your choosing.

Instructions;

- Make sure you have all of the following components on hand: 1 cup of Greek yogurt, 1 tablespoon of honey, and a handful of fresh berries You can use any berries you choose, such as strawberries, blueberries, or raspberries.

- Assemble your yogurt parfait in a bowl or a glass.
- Begin by spooning 1 cup of Greek yogurt into a mixing dish.
- 1 tablespoon honey drizzled over Greek yogurt. Adjust the amount to your preferred sweetness level.
- Place a handful of fresh berries gently on top of the yogurt. Mix several varieties of berries for a colorful and tasty mixture.
- You can keep the layers separate for a more visually pleasing presentation or gently incorporate the honey and berries into the yogurt for a more blended flavor.
- You may now enjoy your Greek yogurt with honey and berries. Enjoy the creamy texture of Greek yogurt, the inherent sweetness of honey, and the crispness of fresh berries in this tasty and nutritious snack or breakfast choice.

Carrot and Cucumber Sticks with Hummus

Ingredients;

- Carrot sticks (1 medium carrot)
- Cucumber sticks (1/2 cucumber)
- Hummus - Use as a dip.

Instructions;

- Prepare the following ingredients: carrot sticks (from 1 medium carrot), cucumber sticks (from 1/2 cucumber), and your favorite hummus for dipping.
- Wash the carrot and cucumber thoroughly. You can peel the carrot if you want. Thinly slice the carrot and cucumber. You can alter the length and thickness of the sticks to suit your needs.
- Arrange the carrot and cucumber sticks on a serving dish or in a small bowl.
- Serve the carrot and cucumber sticks with your preferred hummus. Use the hummus as a pleasant and nutritious dip for the vegetables.

- Carrot and cucumber sticks with hummus create a tasty and healthy snack or appetizer. The brilliant colors and crunchy texture of the vegetables wonderfully complement the creamy and flavorful hummus.

Almonds and Walnuts Mix

Ingredients;

- 1/4 cup of almonds
- 1/4 cup of walnuts

Instructions;

- Assemble the ingredients, which should contain 1/4 cup almonds and 1/4 cup walnuts.
- Take a clean mixing dish or container.
- Put the almonds and walnuts in the container.
- Mix the almonds and walnuts gently. To equally blend them, use a spoon or simply shake the jar.

- You can put the mixture into small snack-sized bags or containers for simple on-the-go access.
- This almond and walnut mixture is a delicious and healthy snack. You may enjoy this nutritious blend whether you're at home, at work, or on the go. The mix of almonds and walnuts produces a pleasing crunch as well as a rich, nutty flavor.
- To improve the flavor, feel free to add a tiny bit of your favorite ingredient, like a dash of cinnamon or a sprinkle of sea salt. If desired, this might give your nut mix a unique twist.

Homemade Trail Mix

Ingredients;

- Almonds (1/4 cup)
- Walnuts (1/4 cup)
- Dried cranberries (1/4 cup)

Instructions;

- Make sure you have all the ingredients ready, which include 1/4 cup each of dried cranberries, walnuts, and almonds.
- Look for a clean, large enough mixing bowl or container to hold all the components together well.
- Add the walnuts, dried cranberries, and almonds to the mixing bowl.
- Once the ingredients are evenly spread, gently stir them together. To guarantee a uniform mixture, you can shake the container or use a spoon.
- You can divide the trail mix into bags or containers that are the size of snacks. Because of this, it is easy to grab for on-the-go eating.
- This wonderful combination of almonds, walnuts, and dried cranberries gives a delightful blend of flavors and textures.
- The almonds and walnuts offer a pleasant crunch, while the dried cranberries add a hint of sweetness. It's an excellent, nutrient-dense snack.

- Feel free to experiment with different components, such as dark chocolate chips, sunflower seeds, or other nuts and dried fruits that you prefer.

Oatmeal with Banana Slices

Ingredients;

- Rolled oats (1/2 cup)
- Banana slices - Add half a banana or as desired.
- Cinnamon (optional) - A pinch for flavor.

Instructions;

- Make sure all the ingredients are prepared, including 1/2 cup rolled oats, sliced banana, and an optional pinch of cinnamon for flavor.
- Place the half cup of rolled oats in a small saucepan or a bowl that is safe to be microwaved.
- Fill it with your favorite beverage. You can use any milk substitute you desire, or even just water or dairy milk. Your

preferred oatmeal consistency will determine how much liquid to use. A good beginning ratio is usually 1 cup liquid to 1/2 cup oats.

- Put a pot on the stovetop over medium heat if you're using one. As the oats cook, constantly stir them with the liquid. Remove them from the fire once they have the consistency you desire.
- If you're using a microwave, cover the bowl with a microwave-safe lid or plate.
- Cook the oats on high for 1-2 minutes, stirring every 30 seconds to prevent overflow. Adjust the cooking time according to the power of your microwave and the thickness of your oats.
- Once your oatmeal is cooked to your preference, add the banana slices. You can stir them into the oats or stack them on top for presentation.
- If you prefer the warm, soothing flavor of cinnamon, put a bit on top of your porridge. This is optional, and the amount can be modified to your liking. u

Sweet Treats for Migraine-Friendly Indulgence

Chia Seed Pudding:

Ingredients;

- Chia seeds (3 tablespoons)
- Almond milk (1 cup)
- Honey (1-2 tablespoons, adjust to taste)
- Fresh berries (e.g., strawberries, blueberries, raspberries) - Use as a topping.

Instructions;

- Prepare the ingredients, which should include 3 tablespoons of chia seeds, 1 cup of almond milk, honey (1-2 tablespoons, adjust to taste), and fresh berries for topping (e.g., strawberries, blueberries, raspberries).
- In a mixing bowl, add 3 tablespoons of chia seeds and 1 cup of almond milk. Stir carefully to disperse the chia seeds evenly.

- Depending on your preference, add 1-2 teaspoons of honey to the mixture. Start with 1 tablespoon and modify as required.
- Stir the chia seed mixture thoroughly to ensure that the honey is properly combined and the chia seeds are uniformly dispersed.
- Place the mixture in a sealed container or individual serving jars. Refrigerate the chia seed pudding mixture for at least 2–3 hours or overnight. This allows the chia seeds to absorb the liquid and form a pudding-like consistency.
- Remove your chia seed pudding from the refrigerator when you're ready to eat it.
- Serve with fresh berries, such as sliced strawberries, blueberries, or raspberries.
- You can be creative with your fruit selections.
- Chia seed pudding is a healthy and tasty breakfast or snack. Enjoy the creamy smoothness and natural sweetness of this delightful delicacy.

Dark Chocolate-Covered Strawberries

Ingredients;

- Dark chocolate (70% cocoa or higher) - Melted for dipping.
- Fresh strawberries - As many as desired.

Instructions;

- Make sure you have all of the ingredients ready, including dark chocolate with at least 70% cocoa or higher (for melting) and fresh strawberries.
- Wash and thoroughly dry the fresh strawberries. Dry strawberries are needed for improved chocolate adhesion.
- Place the dark chocolate in a microwave-safe bowl or a double boiler. If using a microwave, heat the chocolate in 20–30 second increments, stirring after each, until completely melted. If you're using a double boiler, melt the chocolate by turning it continually over simmering water until it's smooth.

- Dip a strawberry into the melted dark chocolate while holding it by the stem or with a toothpick. To ensure that the strawberry is evenly coated with chocolate, rotate it.
- After dipping, set the chocolate-covered strawberry on a piece of parchment paper or a silicone baking mat. This stops the chocolate from adhering.
- Continue dipping the strawberries in the melted dark chocolate and placing them on parchment paper. Depending on your preferences, you can leave some of the strawberries uncovered or completely coat them.
- Allow the dark chocolate-covered strawberries to cool and harden. You may speed things up by putting them in the refrigerator for 15–30 minutes.
- When the chocolate has set, your dark chocolate-covered strawberries are ready to serve. They are a delectable and luxurious delicacy. Enjoy the delicious

blend of sweet, juicy strawberries and creamy dark chocolate.

Chapter 6: Drinks for All Occasions

Cucumber and Mint Infused Water

Ingredients:

- 1 sliced cucumber
- A handful of fresh mint leaves
- A pitcher of water

Instructions:

- Pour some water into a pitcher and add some cucumber slices and fresh mint leaves.
- Place it in the refrigerator and let it steep for a few hours or overnight.
- Serve chilled.

Citrus-Infused Water

Ingredients:

- Sliced citrus fruits (e.g., lemons, limes, and oranges)
- A pitcher of water

Instructions:

- Pour a pitcher of water over sliced citrus fruits.
- Allow it to soak in the refrigerator for a few hours.
- Take pleasure in the zesty and refreshing flavor.

Berry Smoothie

Ingredients:

- 1 cup mixed berries (blueberries, strawberries, raspberries)
- 1/2 banana
- 1/2 cup plain Greek yogurt
- 1 tablespoon honey (optional)
- 1/2 cup almond milk

Instructions:

- Smoothly blend plain Greek yogurt, almond milk, mixed berries, banana, and honey (if using) until well combined.

- To get the desired sweetness and consistency, adjust the components.

Green Smoothie

Ingredients:

- 1 cup fresh spinach
- 1 banana
- 1/2 cup diced apple or pear
- 1/2 cup almond milk
- 1 tablespoon honey (optional)

Instructions:

- Blend fresh spinach, a banana, a sliced apple or pear, almond milk, and honey (if desired) until smooth.
- Adjust the ingredients to suit your taste.

Lemon Ginger Tea

Ingredients:

- 1/2 lemon, freshly squeezed
- 1 teaspoon grated ginger
- A cup of hot water

Instructions:

- In a cup of hot water, mix freshly squeezed lemon juice and grated ginger.
- Allow for a few minutes of steeping before serving.

Conclusion

Finally, "Migraine Relief Kitchen" is your vital guide to adopting a migraine-friendly diet and reclaiming a headache-free life. This book enables you to take responsibility for your migraine management by emphasizing the necessity of identifying and avoiding common migraine triggers, offering a variety of nutritional and balanced meals, proposing mindful snacking techniques, and emphasizing the value of proper hydration.

With the mouthwatering recipes and practical suggestions offered in this book, you'll have the tools you need to develop a healthier relationship with food, reduce migraine episodes, and improve your overall well-being. Remember that every meal is an opportunity to prepare your body against the challenges of migraines and that your journey to a migraine-free life begins here.

Say goodbye to migraines and hello to a brighter, more flavorful future. It's time to relish the taste of a life with fewer headaches, and it all begins with "Migraine Relief Kitchen."